COMBAT KIDNEY DISEASE THROUGH NUTRITIONAL THERAPY

DEDICATION

This book is dedicated to God Almighty who inspired his creature to acquire knowledge and skills to him be praise and also to my Dad for his significant role played in my education attainment.

TABLE OF CONTENTS

DEDICATION	2
CHAPTER ONE	6
Introduction	6
Renal illnesses 'warning signals and symptoms	7
Types of Kidney Diseases	7
CHAPTER TWO	13
Primary Causes of Kidney Disease	13
Symptoms of Glomerulonephritis	16
Glomerulonephritis classification	16
Glomerulonephritis Treatments Kidney Disease	17
Polycystic kidney disease	18
The Origins and Signs of PKD	18
Therapy for PKD	19
CHAPTER THREE	21
Kidney Stones Disease	21
Causes of Kidney Stones	23
Various kidney stones	23

Risk Elements	24
Various Stages of Kidney Diseases	25

CHAPTER FOUR — 28

Healthy Food for Kidney Diseases	28
Foods that are good for renal health	28
Foods Low in Potassium	29
Other Commendable Mentions	29
Foods that Harm Kidney Function	30

CHAPTER FIVE — 32

Nutrition & Dietary for Kidney Disease	32
Heart-healthy Foods	35
Foods Lower in Phosphorus:	36
Foods with less potassium	38
Foods High in Potassium:	38

CHAPTER SIX — 39

Maintaining Fitness despite Kidney Disease	39
Benefits of exercise	40
Prevention Techniques	40

| The benefits of Exercise for Kidney Patients | 41 |

CHAPTER SEVEN | 43

Diabetes Recipes	43
Breakfast:	43
Dinner recipes for Diabetes:	62

Chapter One

Introduction

The kidneys are two important organs that are important to the body. They are in charge of eliminating waste materials and extra fluid from the blood as urine. Additionally, the kidneys create and control the hormones that control blood pressure and promote the creation of red blood cells. Because the early symptoms can be quite faint until the disease is advanced, some people may have kidney disease and be unaware of it. The progression of kidney illness from chronic kidney disease (CKD) to kidney failure can take many years. As the illness worsens, the symptoms become more visible, and the patient starts to experience substantial pain when urinating; if they are even able to urinate at all, the urine may be very black or bloody. Nevertheless, some individuals with the chronic renal disease remain kidney-free their entire lives. Chronic kidney disease is a condition in which the kidneys gradually lose tissue over time.

Kidney disease can cause a wide range of symptoms, some of which are as simple as feeling unwell and weak and others which manifest as infections or kidney stones. However, most people do not often experience symptoms of illness until later stages, when their kidneys are no longer able to filter enough blood each minute.

Renal illnesses 'warning signals and symptoms

- Nausea
- Vomiting
- Reduced appetite
- Weakness and fatigue
- Issues with sleep
- Urinating frequently
- Reduced mental clarity
- Muscle pain
- Swelling in the ankles and feet
- Itchy, dry skin
- Hard to regulate high blood pressure (hypertension)
- Breathlessness if pulmonary fluid accumulates
- Chest discomfort may result If fluid accumulates around the heart's lining,

Types of Kidney Diseases

We place a high value on our kidneys. The occurrence of kidney illness might be disastrous for a person who does not have working kidneys. In the worst situation, dialysis or a kidney transplant will be required to replace the damaged kidneys. Kidney disease can take many various forms, some of which are more severe than others. Kidney disease can be "**chronic**," which denotes a steady deterioration in kidney function, or "**acute**," which denotes a rapid onset. Autoimmune conditions, toxins, drugs, or infections can cause either type of kidney disease. The kidneys' ability to operate can gradually deteriorate due to conditions like diabetes and high blood pressure.

When certain bodily fluids or chemicals escape from the kidneys, renal disease is classified in a different way. Blood in the urine, often known as hematuria, is one of these illnesses. This can happen when the kidneys become unwell and the capillaries in the kidneys begin to leak blood cells. The other is termed proteinuria, and it is pretty typical. Protein leakage from the body, primarily albumin, is known as proteinuria. When this happens, the blood of the remainder of the body may not contain enough protein. Without protein, fluid spills into the body's tissues everywhere because protein keeps the fluid in the blood vessels where it belongs. "Nephrotic syndrome" is the name given to this condition.

Kidney disease can also exist if there are kidney stones. When a person doesn't drink enough water and secretes too much calcium oxalate into the urine, this can happen. As well as kidney stones, uric acid can induce them. When uric acid or calcium oxalate accumulates in the kidneys' urine system, they precipitate into kidney stones that are extremely painful to pass through. Due to their poor fit in the ureters, kidney stones can become lodged there and cause severe pain and a urine backup. Kidney stones can sometimes be accompanied with infections.

Kidney disease can be brought on by hypertension or, less frequently, by the drugs used to treat hypertension (high blood pressure). One or both of the arteries leading to the kidneys may be blocked in some people. In response, the kidneys release vasopressin, which significantly raises blood pressure. There are particular blood pressure medicines that deal with this issue. Surgery may occasionally be required to remove the obstruction.

One other kidney condition is chronic pyelonephritis. Infection can affect one or both kidneys in this illness, which results in chronic pain and inflammation in the kidneys. A kidney infection of this kind may cause hematuria. The most common kidney illness is a malignant condition. One kidney condition that can develop on its own is renal cell carcinoma. The malignancy may result in pain or bleeding near the kidneys. This type of kidney disease may be identified by an abdominal CT scan. If the cancer doesn't spread past the kidney's outer capsule, the kidney can frequently be removed, making the disease very curable.

Genetics can pass down kidney disease. There are several uncommon genetic kidney illnesses that cause blood or protein to flow from the kidneys. These illnesses can occasionally be treated therapeutically, but sometimes the underlying condition requires dialysis or a kidney transplant to be resolved.

It should be mentioned that kidney illness can affect anyone and individuals with chronic renal diseases receive treatment through dialysis or kidney transplantation when medication and dietary modifications are no longer able to control their symptoms. Dialysis is a safe and efficient method of replacing renal function that has been lost; it does not, however, enhance kidney function. However, as soon as the patient begins receiving dialysis, they will see a significant improvement as many of the symptoms will either lessen or go away entirely. Dialysis comes in two flavors: haemodialyzation and peritoneal dialysis.

1. **Haemodialysis**: Is a form of dialysis that removes waste and extra fluid from the blood that has accumulated. The process of haemodialysis involves the passage of blood through soft tubes to a dialysis machine, where it passes through an artificial kidney or dialyzer, a specialized filter. The blood is cleaned and then re-enters the bloodstream.

2. **Peritoneal**: In this case, blood is cleaned within the body rather than being transported to a machine. Dialysate is administered through a flexible tube known as a catheter into the abdomen, where the lining of the stomach (peritoneum) serves as a natural filter. The trash and extra fluid are then expelled from the blood and dissolved in the cleansing agent. After a number of hours, the spent cleansing solution is removed from the abdomen and replaced with new cleansing solution to start the procedure over.

A kidney transplant entails surgically implanting a kidney from one person's body into the body of another person who is suffering from renal failure. It is possible for the kidney to originate from a deceased person or a living donor who may be a sibling, spouse, friend, or someone who desired to donate a kidney to anyone in need of a transplant. The patient will need to take particular drugs after the transplant to prevent the body from rejecting the new kidney. When opposed to dialysis, kidney transplants can extend life and improve quality of life. The patient won't need to undergo dialysis for many hours each week in this situation, nor will they need to adhere to stringent hydration and diet restrictions. All things considered, the patient will feel better and have more freedom.

The phrase "kidney disease," which covers hundreds, if not thousands, of diseases that have an impact on the kidney, is incredibly wide and encompasses a variety of kidney ailments. Depending on the kind of renal illness and the degree of kidney function still present, different consequences may be observed.

The illnesses, signs, or disorders that are impacted by kidney disease complications are secondary conditions, symptoms, or other disorders. The line separating kidney disease consequences from the disease's symptoms is still unclear in several numbers of instances.

Renal failure, anemia, Dialysis-related Amyloidosis (DRA) after dialysis treatment, Vitamin D deficiency, Excessive Serum Phosphorus, Bone Thinning, and Osteoporosis are among the complications of kidney illness that have been reported in numerous sources

But diabetes, both type 1 and type 2, frequently results in renal failure due to kidney disease, which is a typical consequence. In a perfect world, diabetic patients would have their condition well under control and receive regular monitoring from a medical staff knowledgeable about managing the disease. It could ensure that the serious disease consequences are promptly identified and effectively treated. The patient's best interests are served by a collaborative approach to diagnosing and monitoring this disease.

If individuals with diabetes are educated about their condition, comprehend and put into practice the techniques necessary to better control their blood sugar, blood pressure, and cholesterol levels, and receive routine checkups from their healthcare team, they may reduce their risk for complications. Smokers need to stop smoking, and overweight diabetics need to up their modest diet and exercise routines under the advice of a healthcare professional to help them reach a healthier weight.

Chapter Two

Primary Causes of Kidney Disease

Nearly one in every seven persons in the US is affected by kidney disease, often known as renal illness. It may be simpler to take charge of your kidneys' health if you have a rudimentary understanding of the disease's underlying causes. Additionally, if early intervention is possible, there is a higher chance of maintaining kidney function before the condition worsens. Kidney disease can be brought on by a wide range of factors, including:

Diabetes: This is associated with roughly 45% of all occurrences of kidney failure, is the most common cause of this disease. Despite the fact that diabetes is a risk factor, there is no evidence to suggest that all individuals with the condition would eventually experience renal failure. It is important for diabetic patients to take special care of their kidneys by regularly having a microalbumin urine test done to track protein transport and manage blood sugar levels. If you develop kidney disease, your doctor may suggest one of several treatments to help keep this important organ functioning for a longer period of time.

Hypertension: (commonly known as high blood pressure) since hypertension and renal illness are related, it might be challenging to say which condition comes first. It is well recognized that both kidney illnesses like acute or chronic glomerulonephritis and hypertension can affect the kidneys, particularly chronic kidney issues such as chronic pyelonephritis, nephrosclerosis, etc

The glomeruli of the kidneys become inflamed when there is a renal (kidney) issue, such as glomerulonephritis, which is primarily brought on by streptococcal or other infections. Due to the swelling that results from the inflammation, the blood flow to the renal vessels is diminished as a result of this inflammatory process. Renin (an enzyme) is released into the bloodstream because of reduced blood flow. Angiotensinogen, a plasma protein, is now broken down into angiotensin I as a result of the released renin. Angiotensin-converting enzyme (ACE), which is located in the lungs, interacts further with angiotensin I to transform it into angiotensin II. This angiotensin II causes the release of Aldosterone, which boosts the kidneys' ability to reabsorb salt and water, and the constriction of arterioles, which raises both systolic and diastolic blood pressure.

On the other hand, high blood pressure causes renal ischemia (reduced blood flow to the kidneys), which triggers more renin to be released into the bloodstream. As additional angiotensinogen is converted into angiotensin I to continue the cycle, the release of rennin causes a further increase in blood pressure. However, the use of medications known as ACE inhibitors can assist to interrupt this process or reduce the pace at which angiotensin I is converted to angiotensin II, which will help to regulate the hypertension.The kidneys' blood supply is reduced by high blood pressure, a condition known as renal ischemia. If the kidneys are deprived of blood and oxygen for an extended period of time, physiological changes and complications start to take place in them, and they become more vulnerable to infections, there may be recurrent renal infections. Pyelonephritis and nephrosclerosis have a role in this. Nephosclerosis causes the kidneys' arterioles to become even more constricted, which causes more renin to be released, which in turn causes blood pressure to rise once more. If not treated in a timely manner, recurrent renal infection can progress to chronic pyelonephritis and finally kidney failure. Therefore, it is important to treat renal issues as soon as possible in order to prevent hypertension, and to manage hypertension in order to lessen the likelihood of developing renal disease.

Glomerulonephritis: The kidneys' glomeruli are damaged by this condition, also known as glomerular nephritis, which prevents the kidneys from adequately filtering waste materials and extra fluid from your blood. In many nations, glomerulonephritis is the kidney illness that most frequently leads to end-stage renal or kidney disease.

Primary glomerulonephritis is glomerulonephritis that develops on its own. Secondary glomerulonephritis is the term used when the ailment is brought on by another illness, such as systemic lupus erythematosus or diabetes.

Hazards of Glomerulonephritis

Glomerulonephritis frequently has an unknown cause. Your immune system may be having issues as a result. You are more likely to get this disease, though, if you have certain illnesses. They comprise:

- Disorders of the blood or lymphatic systems

 - Amyloidosis

- Diseases of the blood vessels, such as vasculitis

- Cancer

- Diabetes

- Exposure to hazardous substances like hydrocarbon solvents

- IgA nephropathy

- Heart infections, viruses, or strep infections

- Focal segmental glomerulosclerosis

- Lupus nephritis

Symptoms of Glomerulonephritis

Numerous symptoms of glomerulonephritis are possible, and they might alter over time. Blood in the urine or foamy pee are common signs, as well as swelling (edema) in the face, feet, or belly. Additional signs include a general malaise, back or abdominal pain, aches in the joints and muscles, shortness of breath, diarrhea, and fever. In addition to kidney failure, high blood pressure, the nephrotic syndrome, and cardiovascular illnesses, glomerulonephritis can also result in a number of other problems.

Glomerulonephritis classification

This condition has a gradual onset of symptoms, making it first challenging to identify. It's crucial to undergo yearly exams where you offer a urine sample that could reveal early signs of the disease.

A urine test can detect indications such as low red blood cell counts, white blood cell markers of infection or inflammation, or excess protein, a precursor to kidney impairment known as proteinurea or microalbuminurea.

A BUN or creatinine blood serum test may also be advised by your doctor if you have kidney disease. The extent of the glomerulonephritis will need to be determined by imaging tests such as an ultrasound, computerized tomography (CT) scan, or a biopsy if these first tests reveal that your kidneys are damaged.

Glomerulonephritis Treatments Kidney Disease
You must address the underlying condition in secondary glomerular nephritis to prevent further kidney damage. As excessive blood glucose destroys the glomeruli, diabetes is one of the main causes of this kidney condition. Having a successful diabetes control strategy is therefore essential. This can involve the use of suitable natural treatments, such as dietary and lifestyle modifications, as well as herbs and nutrients that help control blood sugar. Glomerulonephritis may go away on its own once the infection has been treated when infections are to blame. Check your blood pressure as well, and if it's high, take action to lower it. Reduced sodium intake, weight loss, increased intake of fruits and vegetables, and supplementation with herbs, garlic, or curcumin are just a few of the natural approaches to lower blood pressure. Blood pressure can also be lowered by a natural diuretic like green tea or dandelion leaf tea. Angiotensin-converting enzyme (ACE) inhibitors, which are available only by prescription, assist in immediately lowering kidney damage.

Polycystic kidney disease

The condition known as "polycystic kidney disease," or "PKD," is inherited and results in the growth of several non-cancerous cysts, which can appear anywhere in the body but most frequently do so in the kidneys. These cysts have the potential to significantly increase kidney size and result in persistent scarring of the normal kidney tissues, impairing kidney function. Due to the lack of symptoms, some people may have this condition for many years without even realizing it, while others may experience very severe symptoms, such as a considerable decline in kidney function or even complete renal failure.

The Origins and Signs of PKD

There are two forms of polycystic kidney disease, and both are brought on by inherited genetic defects. The underlying genetic flaws that led to the two forms of this illness are their main distinctions. The most prevalent type of this condition is "autosomal dominant polycystic kidney disease," or ("ADPKD"). It is typically diagnosed in adults between the ages of thirty and forty; however it can also affect youngsters. If one parent has ADPKD, there is a 50% risk that the child will as well. Due to the requirement that both parents of a child have the defective gene that causes this disease, the other form of PKD, known as "Autosomal recessive Polycystic Kidney Disease" or "ARPKD," is less frequent than ADPKD. There is a 25% probability that a kid may be born with this syndrome if both parents have the faulty gene. The condition known as ARPKD is most frequently identified at birth, although it can also be identified later on in infancy or when the kid has reached puberty. These could be some of the signs of this illness:

- Hypertension (high blood pressure)

- The abdominal region may develop or grow larger.

- Continual urination

- Urine may contain blood.

- Kidney stones could form in a person's body.

- Kidneys or the urinary tract may become infected.

- Because of the expansion of the kidneys, pain may develop in the back around those organs.

- Continual headaches

- Kidney disease (end-stage renal disease)

Therapy for PKD
Treatment for polycystic kidney disease usually entails managing the symptoms or consequences that can result from this condition as there is no known cure for PKD. Patients with renal disease frequently experience high blood pressure; as a result, blood pressure medicines may be administered. Due to their condition, many people have chronic pain. Mild to moderate discomfort may be managed with over-the-counter drugs, but in more serious situations, a doctor may advise surgical excision of larger cysts in order to reduce the agony and pressure that can result.

It is not spreadable; you cannot contract kidney illness from another person. However, some of the main causes, such as diabetes and high blood pressure, can run in families. It is important to get your kidney function, blood sugar, and blood pressure evaluated by your doctor regularly on a regular basis if you have family members who have this condition or know someone who does.

Chapter Three

Kidney Stones Disease

Kidney stones are hard deposits consisting of minerals and salts that develop inside your kidneys. They are also known as renal calculi, nephrolithiasis, or urolithiasis. Kidney stones can be caused by a variety of factors, including diet, excess body weight, and various medical conditions, specific supplements, and drugs. Any section of your urinary tract, from your kidneys to your bladder, might be impacted by kidney stones. When urine becomes concentrated, minerals can crystallize and adhere to one another and frequently lead to stones.

Although passing kidney stones can be extremely painful, if they are caught early enough, they typically don't result in permanent harm. You might only need to take painkillers and drink a lot of water to clear a kidney stone, depending on your circumstances. Surgery might be required in other situations, such as when stones become trapped in the urinary tract, are linked to an infection, or result in problems. If you have a higher chance of getting kidney stones again, your doctor may suggest preventive care to lower your risk.

Until a kidney stone moves around or enters one of the ureters, symptoms are typically not present. The tubes that link the kidneys and bladder are known as ureters. A kidney stone that becomes stuck in the ureters can restrict the urine's flow, inflame the kidney, and cause the ureter to spasm, all of which can be excruciatingly painful. You can then experience the following signs:

- Severe, stabbing pain below the ribcage on the side and back
- Radiating discomfort in the groin and lower abdomen
- Pain that is intermittent and varies in severity
- When urinating, there may be pain or burning.

Other warning signs and symptoms could be:

- Brown, crimson, or pink urine
- cloudy or stench-filled pee
- a constant want to urinate, urinating more frequently than normal, or urinating infrequently
- nausea and diarrhea
- if there are an infection, fever, and chills

As the kidney stone passes through your urinary path, the pain it causes may alter, such as moving to a different spot or becoming more intense. If you experience any signs or symptoms, immediately seek medical help if you experience:

- You are in such much pain that you are unable to remain motionless or find a comfortable position.
- Experiencing pain, nausea, and vomiting
- The presence of pain, fever, and chills
- urine with blood in it
- difficulty urinating

Causes of Kidney Stones

Several factors may raise your risk of developing kidney stones, although there is frequently no one specific explanation.

Kidney stones develop when your urine contains more crystal-forming substances than it can effectively dilute, such as calcium, oxalate, and uric acid. The conditions for kidney stones to form are favorable if your urine lacks chemicals that keep crystals from adhering to one another.

Various kidney stones

Finding out what kind of kidney stone you have can assist identify its source and may provide information on how to lower your risk of developing additional kidney stones. If you pass a kidney stone, attempt to keep it if you can so you may give it to your doctor for analysis.

The following are kidney stone types:

Calcium crystals: Calcium stones, typically in the form of calcium oxalate, make up the majority of kidney stones. Your liver produces oxalate every day, and you can also get it from food. The oxalate level of some fruits, vegetables, nuts, and foods like chocolate is high. The amount of calcium or oxalate in urine can rise due to dietary factors, excessive vitamin D dosages, intestinal bypass surgery, various metabolic illnesses, and dietary factors.

Calcium phosphate: stones are another type of calcium stone that can develop. This kind of stone occurs more frequently in metabolic disorders such as renal tubular acidosis. It might also be connected to several drugs used to treat migraines or seizures, like topiramate (Topamax, Trokendi XR, and Qudexy XR).

Struvite Stones: Urinary tract infections can cause the formation of struvite stones. Sometimes with few symptoms or little warning, these stones have the potential to grow swiftly and become extremely huge.

Uric acid stones: People with chronic diarrhea or malabsorption, those who consume a high protein diet, those who have diabetes or metabolic syndrome, and those who lose too much fluid can all develop uric acid stones. Your risk of uric acid stones may also be increased by specific genetic variables.

Cystine stones: People who have the inherited condition cystinuria, which causes the kidneys to discharge an excessive amount of a particular amino acid, are more likely to develop these stones.

Risk Elements

Your risk of having kidney stones is affected by the following factors:

Personal or family history. You're more likely to get kidney stones if someone in your family has had them. You have a higher chance of getting kidney stones again if you've already had one or more.

Dehydration: Your risk of kidney stones can increase if you don't drink enough water every day. People who sweat a lot and live in warm, dry climates may have a higher risk than others.

Certain diets: Consuming a diet high in sodium (salt), sugar, and protein may raise your chance of developing some kidney stones. This is particularly valid when eating a lot of sodium. Your risk of kidney stones greatly increases when you consume too much salt, which increases the quantity of calcium your kidneys must filter.

Obesity: Kidney stone risk has been associated with a high body mass index (BMI), a large waist, and weight gain.

Surgery and digestive disorders. Changes in the digestive system that influence your absorption of calcium and water might increase the levels of stone-forming chemicals in your urine. These changes can be brought on by gastric bypass surgery, inflammatory bowel disease, or persistent diarrhea.

Your risk of kidney stones might also be increased by other medical diseases such as renal tubular acidosis, cystinuria, hyperparathyroidism, and recurreUTIsuTIs.

Your risk of kidney stones can be increased by taking certain vitamins, supplements, laxatives (when used excessively), calcium-based antacids, and drugs for migraines or depression. Vitamin C is another example.

Various Stages of Kidney Diseases
There are five stages of chronic kidney disease, which vary depending on your age, gender, race, and blood creatinine levels, among other factors. Stage one, when there is a modest variation in filtration rates, is the first stage, and Stage Five, often known as the end stage, is the last. At that time, survival depends on dialysis or organ transplantation.

As was said in the prior post, the stage you are in is determined by your glomerular filtration rate.

Stage 1: A 90 or greater filtration rate. Unless they are tested for anything else and it is found, most people are unaware of this stage.

Stage 2: From 60 to 89, this stage is described as mildly decreasing. The majority of people, like in Stage One, are not aware they have a problem.

Stage 3: From 30 to 59, there is a mild decline. The decline in function is apparent at this time. Anemia and bone loss are both probable, and your blood pressure is likely to increase. You can have constant fatigue, changes in the color and volume of your urine flow, and edema due to fluid retention.

Stage 4: Significant decline, from 16 to 29. The signs and symptoms worsen. You might have a change in taste, an absence of appetite, difficulty sleeping, and trouble concentrating. At this stage, dialysis preparations will probably be recommended.

Stage 5: 15 or less, also known as the end stage. In essence, your kidneys are unable to function. Headaches, pain, cramps in the muscles, nausea, and vomiting are probable. Death is likely without dialysis or a transplant.

Here are a few ideas that will likely be put forth. Most likely, cutting back on sodium will be first on the list. It can cause fluid retention in addition to increasing blood pressure. It's likely that potassium and phosphorus will also be limited. A restriction on protein and hydration intake may be necessary. The disease's progression might be slowed by these modifications.

People are more likely to receive a good diagnosis from their doctor faster if they are more aware of the numerous symptoms and repercussions of being in each stage. The best strategy for effective therapy is early detection.

Puffiness under the eyes, swelling in the ankles and feet, blood in the urine, back pain, burning or difficulty urination, difficulty concentrating and breathing, high blood pressure, nausea, and a metallic taste in the mouth are some of the early symptoms of kidney disease.

If you notice any of these signs, speak with your doctor right away to stop further kidney damage. Blood tests can rule out anomalies in kidney function, so your doctor may recommend them.

Chapter Four

Healthy Food for Kidney Diseases

Your overall health and well-being depend on your kidneys. They are in charge of removing toxins, waste, and surplus fluid from your body. They also control the metabolism of vitamin D, the synthesis of red blood cells, and blood pressure. However, kidney illness is becoming more common. People frequently don't recognize there is issues until their kidneys have suffered serious damage. One method to prevent or treat kidney disease is through a healthy diet. Fill up on meals that improve kidney function and stay away from those that encourage illness.

Foods that are good for renal health
Fish

Although fish is a rich source of protein and it is vital to limit protein intake to protect renal function, it also has additional advantages. Many varieties of fish are healthier sources of protein because they are lower in fat than red meat, pork, or chicken. While other meats are strong in saturated fats, which are hazardous, fatty fish like salmon, mackerel, tuna, and herring are packed with omega-3 essential fatty acids that boost cardiovascular health. You are more susceptible to cardiovascular disease if you have kidney disease. Additionally, studies have shown that fish helps prevent obesity, a key contributor to type 2 diabetes, which is a major cause of kidney disease.

Foods Low in Potassium

Along with sodium and phosphorus, potassium is a mineral that you should decrease to enhance kidney function. Though potassium is present in a wide range of meals, its presence is less obvious than that of salt or sugar, for example, because you cannot taste potassium. Try to stick to low-potassium foods like tangerines, cucumbers, summer squash, blackberries, grapes, pears, onions, asparagus, cabbage, and cauliflower. Additionally, look for potassium content on food items.

Leaf Tea

Antioxidants found in abundance in this well-known beverage shield organs, particularly the kidneys, from infection and free radical damage. Additionally, kidney stones, which can harm the kidneys, might be avoided.

Green Tea

Green tea also contains anti-inflammatory qualities, and enhances cardiovascular health, including lowering cholesterol levels and preventing atherosclerosis, according to the University of Maryland Medical Center in the United States. It also acts as a natural diuretic and aids in removing extra fluid from the body, a process that is hampered when the kidneys aren't functioning properly.

Other Commendable Mentions

- Black beans

- Asparagus
- Watermelon
- Celery

Foods that Harm Kidney Function
Protein

The quantity of nitrogen-containing amino acids that must be expelled in urine as urea can be reduced by limiting your protein consumption. These toxins accumulate in your blood when your kidneys aren't working properly, harming the filtering of the blood vessels in the kidneys.

Start by cutting back on the amount of meat and dairy products you consume. Change them out for more wholesome sources like soy, whole grains, seafood, and occasionally low-fat fowl.

Processed and quick meals

These foods are high in salt, which you should avoid if you want to improve kidney health and treat renal disease. They typically include high levels of phosphates. Phosphates influence bone health, which is already at risk if you have a renal illness because vitamin D metabolism is affected, as well as the protein and nitrogen balances in the body.

Oily foods

The risk of cardiovascular disorders including heart attacks and stroke increases as a result of kidney disease. Triglyceride and cholesterol levels are also raised by fatty diets. Fatty meals encourage weight gain and raise your risk of getting diabetes, one of the main causes of kidney disease, by raising the level of fat in your body.

As you can see, even a few little dietary adjustments can help to protect your kidneys from harm, and nutritional supplements have even been proven to be effective at treating renal disease.

Chapter Five

Nutrition & Dietary for Kidney Disease

To manage renal illness, you might need to alter your diet. Develop a meal plan that incorporates items you like to eat while preserving the health of your kidneys with the help of a registered dietitian. You can control your kidney illness by following the guidelines below, which will help you eat healthily. For everyone who has kidney disease, the first three steps (1-3) are crucial. As the function of your kidneys declines, the final two steps (4-5) may become crucial.

The very first steps to eating healthy:

Step 1: Select and cook foods with less salt and sodium

Why? to assist in blood pressure management. Less than 2,300 mg of sodium per day ought to be included in your diet. Frequently purchase fresh food. Many prepared or packaged foods you purchase at the grocery store or in restaurants have sodium (a component of salt) added. Instead of consuming prepared, "fast," frozen, and canned foods that are higher in sodium, cook your meals from scratch. You decide what goes into your food when you make it.

Replace salt with spices, herbs, and seasonings without sodium.

Look for sodium on the Nutrition Facts label on food containers. The food is high in sodium if it has a Daily Value of 20% or more.

Consider frozen dinners and other convenience items in lower-sodium varieties. Before eating, rinse canned fish, meats, and vegetables with water.

Look for words on food labels like "salt-free" "sodium-free," "low," "reduced," or "no salt," as well as "unsalted" or "lightly salted."

An illustration of a nutrition facts product label showing a 5% daily value for salt in a serving.

Check the food label for salt content. The sodium content of a food is minimal if the Percent Daily Value is 5% or below. Additionally, check the label to see how much saturated and trans fats are there.

Step 2: Consume the appropriate amounts and varieties of protein.

Yes? to support the kidneys' protection. Your body generates waste when it consumes protein. This waste is removed by your kidneys. Your kidneys may have to work harder if you consume more protein than you require.

Eat protein-rich foods in moderation.

Foods made from both plants and animals include protein. Both sources of protein are typically consumed. Consult a nutritionist for advice on the best protein food combinations for you.

Foods with animal protein:

Chicken

Fish

Meat

Eggs

Dairy

Approximately 2 to 3 ounces, or roughly the size of a deck of cards, make up a cooked serving of chicken, fish, or meat. A serving of dairy products is equal to one slice of cheese, yogurt, or half a cup of milk.

Plant-based proteins:

Nuts

Beans

Grains

A piece of nuts is equal to one-quarter cup, and a quantity of cooked beans is roughly one-half cup. A serving of cooked rice or cooked noodles is equal to one-half cup, and a serving of bread is one slice.

Step 3: Select heart-healthy meals to eat.

Why? to prevent the accumulation of fat in your kidneys, heart, and blood vessels.

Replace deep frying with grilling, broiling, baking, roasting, or stir-frying.

Instead of using butter for cooking, use nonstick cooking spray or a small amount of olive oil.

Before eating, trim the fat from the meat and take the skin from the chicken.

Limit your intake of saturated and trans fats. Go over the food label.

Heart-healthy Foods
Lean meat cuts, like loin or round Poultry without the skin

Fish

Beans

Vegetables

Fruits

Milk, yogurt, and cheese that are low-fat or fat-free. To help safeguard your blood vessels, heart, and kidneys, chooses heart-healthy foods.

Restrict your alcohol consumption.

Only consume alcohol in moderation; no more than one drink for women per day and no more than two for men. Alcoholism is a major health risk factor that can harm the liver, heart, and brain. How much alcohol is safe for you to consume? Ask your healthcare practitioner.

The subsequent steps to healthy eating,

You might need to consume fewer foods high in phosphorus and potassium as your kidney function declines. Your doctor will use lab tests to check the levels of potassium and phosphorus in your blood, and you can work with a dietitian to modify your diet.

Step 4: Pick phosphorus-free foods and beverages,

The reason? to aid in preserving your blood vessels and bones. Phosphorus can build up in your blood when you have CKD. Your bones become thin, weak, and more prone to breaking when your blood phosphorus level is too high because it removes calcium from them. Additionally, to causing itchy skin, high blood phosphorus levels can also hurt your bones and joints. Phosphorus is frequently added to packaged meals. Look for words with "PHOS" or the word "phosphorus" on ingredient labels. Phosphorus may be added to deli meats, some fresh meats, and some fowl. Request assistance from the butcher in choosing fresh meats free of added phosphorus.

Foods Lower in Phosphorus:
Fresh fruits and vegetables

Breads, pasta, rice

Rice milk (not enriched)

Corn and rice cereals

Light-colored sodas/pop, such as lemon-lime or homemade iced tea

Foods Higher in Phosphorus:

Meat, poultry, fish

Bran cereals and oatmeal

Dairy foods

Beans, lentils, nuts

Several bottled or canned iced teas with additional phosphorus, fruit punch, and dark-colored sodas/pop-top reduce the quantity of phosphorus in your blood; your doctor may suggest taking a phosphate binder with meals. A phosphate binder is a medication that absorbs or binds phosphorus in the stomach in a similar manner to a sponge. The phosphorous does not enter your bloodstream since it is bonded. The phosphorous is instead eliminated by your body through stools.

Step 5: Pick foods that have the proper amount of potassium

Why? to promote proper nerve and muscle function. Too much or too little potassium in the blood might cause issues. Potassium can build up in your blood as a result of damaged kidneys, which can seriously harm your heart. If necessary, you can lower your potassium level by choosing certain foods and beverages.

Potassium levels in salt substitutes can be very high. Examine the ingredient list. The use of salt replacements should be discussed with your physician.

Fruits and vegetables in cans should be drained before consumption.

Foods with less potassium:

Peaches and apples

Green beans and carrots

Spaghetti and white bread

White rice

Rice milk (not enriched)

Grits, cooked rice, and wheat cereals

Cranberry, apple, or grape juice

Foods High in Potassium:
Orange juice, bananas, and oranges

Tomatoes with potatoes

Wild and brown rice

Grains with bran

Milk products

Whole-wheat pasta and bread

Nuts and beans

Some drugs may also cause an increase in potassium levels. The medications you take may be changed by your healthcare professional.

Chapter Six

Maintaining Fitness despite Kidney Disease

The safety of exercise for those with chronic renal disease has come under scrutiny. Physical activity is recommended by a recent study for people managing impaired renal function. Exercise has been demonstrated to be one of the most effective treatments for kidney illness, as diet slows the course of renal failure (symptomatic relief). According to the study, these patients' health and quality of life can indeed be enhanced by a well-planned exercise regimen.

Exercise is safe, but there are a few things you should watch out for. Additionally, there are some activities that people with renal disease are not supposed to perform. We have covered both of the below topics.

Reasons for Less Physical Activity

Loss of fitness is one of kidney disease's most obvious side effects. The performance of routine chores is extremely tough for people. There are several causes for it. Diets for chronic kidney disease place a range of restrictions on food intake, including calorie and nutrient limits. The muscles are readily worn out. There is a persistent sense of exhaustion. Cramps and jerks in the muscles make the issue worse. A person also struggles to focus and concentrate on the activities at hand.

Benefits of exercise
Patients with CKD are advised to engage in weight training and aerobic exercises. Exercise options include resistance training, aerobic exercise, or a combination of both. Yoga is a healthy type of exercise as well.

The benefits of regular exercise are numerous for the body. It increases metabolic rate and aids in fat burning. As a result, it helps people stay at a healthy weight. Starting to exercise may also cause one's appetite to grow. The muscles are made stronger by resistance exercise, which also increases stamina and endurance. Lethargy is eliminated, and you experience an increase in energy. It raises productivity.

The body consumes more oxygen while it is engaged in aerobic activity. It has been demonstrated to control lipid profiles and blood pressure. Exercises that condition the heart's muscles are cardiovascular inin nature. Enhancing attention and concentration first, and then lowering anxiety and depression second, supports mental health and psychological well-being.

Exercise generally enhances performance. It might help postpone the requirement for dialysis. Additionally, by monitoring lifestyle conditions including diabetes, high blood pressure, and obesity, the risk of total kidney failure is decreased.

Prevention Techniques
Before beginning an exercise program, you should speak with your doctor. If you exercise frequently and have just received a diagnosis of chronic kidney disease, talk to your

doctor about your present regimen. Based on your health, he will assess your present exercise regimen and recommend any required adjustments.

• People on dialysis have different exercise regimens than people who merely take medicine.

• If you stopped working out following your diagnosis and now want to start again, t out slowly and with your doctor first. This will shield you from needless harm and let you keep up your healthy exercise routine.

• You shouldn't strain the body beyond what it can handle.

• You'll be asked by the dietitian to keep an eye on your urine production. He would advise you to drink more fluids to stay hydrated if you perspire.

In the modern environment, physical fitness is essential. A stronger body and better health care benefits that everyone is enjoying. Your body remains robust and healthy with exercise. Exercise makes it simpler to move around, do your important responsibilities, and yet have enough energy left over for other enjoyable activities.

The benefits of Exercise for Kidney Patients
Exercise has a number of advantages than just giving you more energy.

Physical performance of the muscles has improved

Increased control over blood pressure

Better muscular power

Decreased blood lipid levels (cholesterol and triglycerides)

Enhanced slumber

More effective body weight management

Yes. Do not start any fitness program without consulting your doctor beforehand.

Four factors need to be considered when creating a directed exercise program:

Exercise form

How long you spend working out

How frequently you work out

How difficult an exercise is.

Fitness Activity for Kidney Patient

Select activities that need you to move your muscles continuously, such as walking, swimming, biking (indoors or outdoors), skiing, aerobic dance, or any other such activity.

Low-intensity strengthening exercises could be a helpful addition to your regimen. Create a program using light weights and lots of repetitions, and steer clear of heavy lifting.

Chapter Seven

Diabetes Recipes

Breakfast:

- **Sandwiches made with eggs, tomatoes, and feta:**

Egg sandwiches with tomato, feta, and rosemary

These filling breakfast sandwiches are loaded with feta, tomato, and spinach-ingredients that are common in Mediterranean cooking.

Active: Five mins

Total: Twenty mins

Servings: Four

Ingredients

Four multigrain thin sandwiches

Olive oil, four tablespoons

One-half teaspoon crushed dried rosemary or one tablespoon freshly chopped rosemary

Four eggs

Two cups of young, fresh spinach leaves

One medium tomato thinly sliced into eight pieces.

Four tablespoons of feta cheese with little fat

One-eighth kosher salt spoon

Black pepper freshly ground

Local Deals

Directions:

Step one

Set oven to 375 degrees Fahrenheit. Sandwich thins should be split; brush the sliced sides with 2 teaspoons of olive oil. Place on a baking sheet and toast for five minutes, or until crisp and light brown around the edges.

Step two

In the meantime, heat the rosemary and the remaining two tablespoons of olive oil in a large skillet over medium-high heat. One at a time, crack eggs into the skillet. Cook for approximately a minute, or until the yolks are still runny but the whites are set. Use a spatula to crack the yolks. Flip eggs over and continue to cook until done. Get rid of the heat.

Step three

On four serving plates, arrange the bottom halves of the toasted sandwich thins. Sandwich thins on platters should all have spinach on them. Add two tomato slices, one egg, and one tablespoon of feta cheese to the top of each. Add little pepper and salt to taste. Add the last of the thin sandwich halves on top.

Nutritional Facts

One sandwich per serving, serving size: 242 calories; 13g protein; 25g crabs; 6.2g dietary fiber; sugars; 11.7g fat; 2.9g saturated fat; 214mg cholesterol; 2448.4IU vitamin A; 12mg vitamin C; 28.7mcg folate; 123.2mg calcium; 3mg iron; 9.9mg magnesium; 143.8mg potassium; and 501.2mg sodium.

- **Banana pancakes with only two ingredients**

Best enjoyed immediately after cooking, these pancakes are delicious and incredibly easy to make. Healthy grain-free pancakes with no added sugar can be made with simply eggs and a banana. Yogurt or ricotta cheese can be served with maple syrup to add some protein.

Active: Ten mins.

Total: Ten mins.

Servings: Two

Ingredients:

Two huge eggs.

One medium banana

Directions:

Step one

Bananas and eggs should be blended to a smooth consistency.

Step two

Over medium heat, lightly oil a sizable nonstick skillet (see Tip). Four mounds of batter should be poured into the skillet, with two tablespoons of batter for each pancake. Two to four minutes of cooking time is enough to get surface bubbles and dry-looking edges. Gently flip the pancakes with a thin spatula and continue cooking for an additional one to two minutes or until the bottoms are golden. Onto a platter, place the pancakes. Repeat with the remaining batter, re-lightly lubricating the pan.

Tips Tip: To lightly oil a nonstick pan, blot a piece of crumpled paper towel with oil and wipe the oil over the skillet's surface.

Nutritional Facts

The serving size is four pancakes. 124 calories; 6.9 grams of protein; 13.8, 1.5 grams of carbohydrates; sugars; 4.9 grams of fat; 1.6 grams of saturated fat; 186 mg of cholesterol; 307.8 IU of vitamin A; 5.1 mg of vitamin C; 35.3 mg of folate; 31 milligrams of calcium; 1 milligram of iron; 21.9 milligrams of magnesium; 280.2 milligrams of potassium; and 71.6 milligrams of sodium.

Exchanges: One fruit for one medium-fat protein.

- **Pineapple-Grapefruit Detox Smoothie**

The water and minerals found in spinach, pineapple, and grapefruit can help hydrate you and provide a wealth of fiber for your body. A cooling dairy-free alternative to yogurt or milk is electrolyte-rich coconut water. For an extra-frozen smoothie, freeze the coconut water into cubes if you have the time.

Active: Ten mins

Total: Ten mins

Servings: Two

Ingredients:

One cup unsweetened coconut water

One cup of diced frozen pineapple

One cup of baby spinach, packed

One small grapefruit, peeled and segmented, along with any membrane juice

Grated fresh ginger, half a teaspoon

Ice, one cup

Directions:

Step one

Blend coconut water, ginger, ice, pineapple, spinach, grapefruit, and any liquids. Purée until foamy and smooth.

Nutritional Facts

Around one and a half cups per serving

Each Serving: vitamin an in 2808.2IU, vitamin c 94mcg, folate 78.2mcg, calcium 58mg, iron 1.3mg, magnesium 45.5mg, potassium 433.1mg, sodium 54.4mg, and thiamin 0.1mg. 102 calories; 2g protein; 2g crabs; 2.9g dietary fiber; sugars 19.9g; and 0.2g fat.

One and a half fruit is substituted.

- **A hearty oatmeal recipe with tomato and sausage.**

In this delicious recipe, oats are given new life as the base for a pleasing combination of sausage, greens, tomatoes, and herbs.

Active: Ten mins.

Total Fifteen mins

.Servings: One

Two tablespoons of canola or sunflower oil, split

Sweet Italian chicken sausage (half link) weighing one and a half ounces when fully cooked

Old-fashioned rolled oats and one cup of low-sodium vegetable broth

A salt shaker full

Halves of a cup of grape tomatoes

One-third cup of fresh herbs, like cilantro and/or parsley, that have been packed

Twelve cups of packed baby arugula

Pine nuts, roasted, one tablespoon (see Tip)

A sizable wedge of lemon

Directions:

Step one

A small cast-iron or nonstick skillet should be heated over medium heat with one teaspoon of oil. Ten minutes or so later, add the sausage and cook it thoroughly.

Step two

In the meantime, in a small pan over high heat, bring the broth to a boil. Oats and salt are added after stirring. The heat is then reduced to medium, and the mixture is cooked for about five minutes, with periodic stirring.

Step three

Cut the sausage into coins with a razor blade. Oatmeal has been cooked; add the sausage, tomatoes, and seasonings. to a bowl, transfer. Sprinkle the remaining one tsp. of oil over the top and add the arugula and pine nuts. Optimally, serve with a wedge of lemon.

Tips Tip: To toast pine nuts, place them in a small, dry skillet over medium-low heat and cook, turning regularly, for two to four minutes, or until aromatic. Let cool after transferring to a small plate.

Nutritional Facts

Serving Size: two and one quarter cups Per Serving: 391 calories; 15g protein; 36g crabs; 7g dietary fiber; 6g sugars; 22g fat; 3g saturated fat; 33mg cholesterol; 535mg potassium; and 689mg sodium.

- **Authentic Green Smoothie**

This nutritious smoothie recipe is very green because it contains both kale and avocado. Chia seeds add a heart-healthy dose of fiber and omega-3 fatty acids to this creamy smoothie.

Active: Five mins

Total Five mins

Servings: One

Ingredients

One substantial ripe banana

One cup mature kale that has been roughly chopped or packed baby kale

One cup of vanilla almond milk without sugar

One quarter ripe avocado

Chia seeds, one tablespoon

Honey, two teaspoons

ice cubes in a cup

Directions:

Step one

In a blender, combine the banana, kale, almond milk, avocado, chia seeds, and honey. Blend at a high speed until smooth and creamy. Blend in ice till smooth.

Nutritional Facts

Serving Size: Two and one-third cups Per Serving: 343 calories; 5.9 grams of protein; 54.7 grams of carbohydrates; 12.1 grams of dietary fiber; 28.8 grams of sugars; 14.2 grams of fat; 1.6 grams of saturated fat; 2264.5 IU of vitamin A; 36.3 mg of folate; 309.6 mg of calcium; 2.1 mg of iron; 112.2 mg of magnesium; 1051.1 mg of potassium; and 198.9 mg of sodium.

Exchanges: three fat, two fruits, one other type of carbohydrate, and one vegetable.

- **Breakfast Salad with Egg & Salsa Verde Vinaigrette**

Salad for breakfast? Don't knock it until you've tried it. We love how this meal gives you 3 whole cups of vegetables to start your day.

Active: Ten mins

Total: Ten mins

Servings: One

Ingredients

Three tablespoons salsa verde, such as Frontera brand

One tablespoon plus one tsp. extra-virgin olive oil, divided

Two tablespoons chopped cilantro, plus more for garnish

Two cups mesclun or other salad greens

Eight blue corn tortilla chips, broken into large pieces

Half cup canned red kidney beans, rinsed

One quarter avocado, sliced

One large egg

Directions:

Step One

Whisk salsa, One Tbsp. oil, and cilantro in a small bowl. Toss half the mixture with mesclun (or other greens) in a shallow dinner bowl.

Step two

Layer chips, beans, and avocado atop the salad.

Step three

Heat the remaining one tsp. oil in a small nonstick skillet over medium-high heat. Add egg and fry until the white is completely cooked but the yolk is still slightly runny, about two minutes.

Step four

Serve the egg on the salad. Drizzle with the remaining salsa vinaigrette and sprinkle with additional cilantro, if desired.

Nutrition Facts

Serving Size: Three cups salad plus one egg plus five Tbsp. vinaigrette

Per Serving: 527 calories; protein 16g; carbohydrates 37g; dietary fiber 13g; sugars 2g; fat 34g; saturated fat 5g; cholesterol 186mg; potassium 1001mg; sodium 660mg.

- **Strawberry-Pineapple Smoothie**

Blend almond milk, strawberry and pineapple for a smoothie that's so easy you can make it on busy mornings. A bit of almond butter adds richness and filling protein. Freeze some of the almond milk for an extra-icy texture.

Active: Five mins

Total: Five mins

Servings: One

Ingredients

One cup frozen strawberries

One cup chopped fresh pineapple

Three-fourths cup chilled unsweetened almond milk, plus more if needed

One tablespoon almond butter

Directions:

Step one

Combine strawberries, pineapple, almond milk and almond butter in a blender. Process until smooth, adding more almond milk, if needed, for desired consistency. Serve immediately.

Nutrition Facts

Serving Size: Two cups

Per Serving: 255 calories; protein 5.6g; carbohydrates 39g; dietary fiber 7.8g; sugars 24g; fat 11.1g; saturated fat 1.1g; vitamin a iu 537.9IU; vitamin c 140.3mg; folate 63.5mcg; calcium 438.3mg; iron 2.4mg; magnesium 80.8mg; potassium 546.3mg; sodium 168.4mg; thiamin 0.2mg.

Exchanges: Two and a half fruit, two fat

- **Avocado-Egg Toast**

Try it once and we think you'll agree: Topping avocado toast with an egg is a near-perfect breakfast.

Active: Five mins

Total: Five mins

Servings: One

Avocado Toast Tips Start with Good Bread

Good avocado toast starts with good bread. Multigrain or whole-wheat bread adds another layer of flavor (and additional fiber) to your avocado toast. Sandwich bread, as well as crusty artisan bread, are both great options. Just make sure the bread is sliced thick enough to hold up to the toppings.

Find the Perfect Avocado

Soft, ripe avocados are perfect for mashing and perfect for your best avocado toast. A perfectly ripe avocado will give to slight pressure, but not feel mushy. You can always cut into your avocado if you are unsure. Some small blemishes in the flesh are ok, just remove them before mashing. If your avocado is very brown, or very soft, it may be past its prime. Conversely, an avocado that is under ripe will be hard to mash and leave you with a lumpy result.

Here's more about finding the perfect avocado.

Give Some TLC to Your Avocado Mash

Simply adding a pinch of salt and pepper can enhance the flavor of your avocado mash, but it doesn't have to stop there. You can jazz it up with chopped fresh herbs, dried spices like garlic powder or chili powder or lime juice for a little tang.

What to Put on Avocado Toast

We top this avocado toast with a fried egg, but the sky is the limit on what you can use to top your toast. Eggs work well for breakfast, as do thinly sliced tomatoes or smoked salmon as a different spin on a cream cheese and lox bagel. Try adding veggies like cucumber, sprouts or salad greens to give your avocado toast a more lunch-like vibe. And of course, you can add a flavorful drizzle like Sriracha, balsamic glaze or salsa to finish it off.

Is Avocado Toast Healthy?

Avocado toast fits perfectly into a healthy diet. Avocados deliver fiber and a dose of healthy fats that help keep your heart healthy and you feeling full for longer periods of time. Pair that with even more fiber-boosting foods like whole-wheat or multigrain toast and the benefits only increase. Diets high in fiber are associated with the prevention of heart disease, diabetes and certain types of cancer.

Ingredients

One-quarter avocado

One-quarter teaspoon ground pepper

One-eighth teaspoon garlic powder

One slice whole-wheat bread, toasted

One large egg, fried

One teaspoon Sriracha (Optional)

One tablespoon scallion, sliced (Optional)

Directions:

Step one

Combine avocado, pepper and garlic powder in a small bowl and gently mash.

Step two

Top toast with the avocado mixture and fried egg. Garnish with Sriracha and scallion, if desired.

Nutrition Facts

Serving Size: One toast

Per Serving: 271 calories; protein 11.5g; carbohydrates 18.1g; dietary fiber 5.4g; sugars 2g; fat 17.7g; saturated fat 3.5g; cholesterol 186mg; vitamin a iu 347.5IU; vitamin c 5mg; folate 77.5mcg; calcium 69.4mg; iron 2mg; magnesium 46.6mg; potassium 406.5mg; sodium 216.2mg.

- **Peanut Butter-Banana English Muffin**

Peanut butter and banana is the original power couple. Top a simple toasted English muffin with the duo, then sprinkle everything with a hit of ground cinnamon for a healthy breakfast of champions.

Active: Five mins

Total: Five mins

Servings: One

Ingredients:

One whole-wheat English muffin, toasted

One tablespoon peanut butter

Half banana, sliced

Pinch of ground cinnamon

Directions:

Step one

Top English muffin with peanut butter, banana and cinnamon.

Nutrition Facts

Serving Size: One serving

Per Serving: 344 calories; protein 10.6g; carbohydrates 56.8g; dietary fiber 8.6g; sugars 20.3g; fat 9.8g; saturated fat 1.6g; vitamin a iu 79.3IU; vitamin c 10.3mg; folate 56mcg; calcium 182.4mg; iron 2.1mg; magnesium 78.8mg; potassium 561.7mg; sodium 293.9mg; added sugar 5g.

Exchanges: One and a half starch, one and a half high-fat protein, one fruit

- **Scrambled Eggs with Sausage**

Start your day off right with these scrambled eggs. This recipe includes eggs, turkey sausage, and cheese; packing fourteen grams of protein per serving. Quick and easy to make, this is the perfect breakfast solution.

Active: Five mins

Total: Ten mins

Servings: Two

Ingredients:

Nonstick cooking spray

Two eggs

Two tablespoons reduced-sodium chicken broth

Ground black pepper

One ounce cooked turkey sausage, sliced

One-quarter cup cherry tomatoes, quartered

Two tablespoons finely shredded reduced-fat Cheddar cheese

One whole-grain English muffin, halved and toasted

Directions:

Step one

Coat a large nonstick skillet with cooking spray. Preheat skillet over medium heat.

Step two

In a medium bowl, use a whisk or rotary beater to beat together eggs, broth and black pepper; stir in sliced sausage.

Step three

Pour egg mixture into hot skillet. Cook over medium heat, without stirring, until mixture begins to set on the bottom and around edges.

Step four

With a spatula or a large spoon, lift and fold the partially cooked egg mixture so the uncooked portion flows underneath. Continue cooking over medium heat until almost set; add tomatoes and cheese. Cook about 1 minute more or until egg mixture is cooked through but is still glossy and moist.

Step five

Serve over toasted English muffin halves.

Nutrition Facts

Serving Size: One English muffin half and one and a half cups egg mixture

Per Serving: 198 calories; protein 14.5g; carbohydrates 15.6g; dietary fiber 2.5g; sugars 4.3g; fat 9.3g; saturated fat 3.1g; cholesterol 230.5mg; vitamin a iu 507.8IU; vitamin c 2.9mg; folate 44.3mcg; calcium 222mg; iron 2.1mg; magnesium 38.5mg; potassium 244.4mg; sodium 523.7mg.

Exchanges: One and a half medium-fat protein, one starch

- **Cherry Smoothie**

The combination of oat milk, vanilla extract and sweet cherries makes this recipe taste like a cherry pie smoothie. Adding a bit of brown sugar boosts that nostalgia even more.

Active: Five mins

Total: Five mins

Servings: One

Ingredients:

Half cup oat milk

One tablespoon almond butter

One teaspoon cocoa powder

Half teaspoon vanilla extract

One cup frozen dark sweet cherries

One tablespoon brown sugar (Optional)

Directions:

Step one

Add oat milk, almond butter, cocoa, vanilla, cherries and sugar (if using) to a blender. Blend until smooth.

Nutrition Facts

Serving Size: One and a half cups

Per Serving: 232 calories; protein 5.7g; carbohydrates 31.5g; dietary fiber 5.8g; sugars 21g; fat 9.1g; saturated fat 1.2g; vitamin a iu 100.2IU; vitamin c 9mg; folate 9.1mcg; calcium 307.8mg; iron 1.5mg; magnesium 53.6mg; potassium 242mg; sodium 86.7mg; added sugar 2g.

Dinner recipes for Diabetes:

- **Chicken & Spinach Skillet Pasta with Lemon & Parmesan**

This one-pan chicken pasta combines lean chicken breast and sautéed spinach for a one-bowl meal that's garlicky, lemony and best served with a little Parm on top. I call it "Mom's Skillet Pasta" and she called it "Devon's Favorite Pasta." Either way it's a quick and easy weeknight dinner we created together and scribbled on a little recipe card more than a decade ago, or it remains in my weekly dinner rotation to this day. It's a simple dinner the whole family will love.

Active: Twenty five mins.

Total: Twenty five mins.

Servings: Four

How to Make Chicken & Spinach Skillet Pasta with Lemon & Parmesan

This chicken pasta dinner is a family-friendly weeknight favorite. Made in just one skillet, clean-up is a breeze.

1) Start the Pasta

To get this dinner on the table fast, get the pasta cooking first. We call for penne pasta but any shape will work. If you have gluten sensitivity, gluten-free pasta works well here. If not, using whole-wheat pasta will give you a boost of fiber without taking away from the flavor of the dish. Make sure not to overcook the pasta which can make the dish mushy at the end.

2) Cook the Chicken

While the pasta cooks, start the chicken. (You will want a high-sided skillet here or a large pot big enough to hold all of the ingredients.) You can use chicken breast or chicken thighs in this recipe. Chicken breast is the better choice if you want a leaner dish with less trimming. Chicken thoughts offer a meatier flavor, but usually need to be trimmed. Make sure the pieces are cut about the same size so they cook evenly.

3) Finish the Dish

Once the chicken is cooked through, you finish the dish by making the sauce! Garlic adds a savory baseline flavor. Wine and lemon juice (and zest) is added to make the sauce bright and tangy. Bringing the sauce to a simmer helps meld the flavors and gets the pan hot enough to rewarm the pasta and wilt the spinach which is added at the end. This dish is at its best served right away sprinkled with Parmesan cheese. Enjoy!

Ingredients:

Eight ounces gluten-free penne pasta or whole-wheat penne pasta

Two tablespoons extra-virgin olive oil

One pound boneless, skinless chicken breast or thighs, trimmed, if necessary, and cut into bite-size pieces

Half teaspoon salt

One-quarter teaspoon ground pepper

Four cloves garlic, minced

Half cup dry white wine

Juice and zest of one lemon

Ten cups chopped fresh spinach

Four tablespoons grated Parmesan cheese, divided

Directions:

Step one

Cook pasta according to package directions. Drain and set aside.

Step two

Meanwhile, heat oil in a large high-sided skillet over medium-high heat. Add chicken, salt and pepper; cook, stirring occasionally, until just cooked through, five to seven minutes. Add garlic and cook, stirring, until fragrant, about One minute. Stir in wine, lemon juice and zest; bring to a simmer.

Step three

Remove from heat. Stir in spinach and the cooked pasta. Cover and let stand until the spinach is just wilted. Divide among four plates and top each serving with one tablespoon Parmesan.

Nutrition Facts

Serving Size: scant two cups

Per Serving: 335 calories; protein 28.7g; carbohydrates 24.9g; dietary fiber 2g; sugars 1.1g; fat 12.3g; saturated fat 2.7g; cholesterol 66.9mg; vitamin a in 7100IU; vitamin c 30.8mg; folate 154.8mcg; calcium 143.6mg; iron 3.3mg; magnesium 107.9mg; potassium 684.5mg; sodium 499.2mg; thiamin 0.2mg.

Exchanges: Three lean protein, two fats, one starch, one vegetable

- **Slow-Cooker Braised Beef with Carrots & Turnips**

The spice blend in this healthy beef stew recipe--cinnamon, allspice and cloves--may conjure images of apple pie, but the combo is a great fit in savory applications too. Serve over creamy polenta or buttered whole-wheat egg noodles.

Active: Forty mins

Total: Four hrs

Servings: Eight

Ingredients:

One tablespoon kosher salt

Two teaspoons ground cinnamon

Half teaspoon ground allspice

Half teaspoon ground pepper

One-quarter teaspoon ground cloves

Three-three and half pounds beef chuck roast, trimmed

Two tablespoons extra-virgin olive oil

One medium onion, chopped

Three cloves garlic, sliced

One cup red wine

One (Twenty eight ounce) cans whole tomatoes, preferably San Marzano

Five medium carrots cut into One-inch pieces

Two medium turnips, peeled and cut into half-inch pieces

Chopped fresh basil for garnish

Directions:

Step one

Combine salt, cinnamon, allspice, pepper and cloves in a small bowl. Rub the mixture all over beef.

Step two

Heat oil in a large skillet over medium heat. Add the beef and cook until browned, 4 to 5 minutes per side. Transfer to a five- to six-quart slow cooker.

Step three

Add onion and garlic to the pan. Cook, stirring, for 2 minutes. Add wine and tomatoes (with their juice); bring to a boil, scraping up any browned bits and breaking up the tomatoes. Add the mixture to the slow cooker along with carrots and turnips.

Step four

Cover and cook on High for 4 hours or Low for 8 hours.

Step five

Remove the beef from the slow cooker and slice. Serve the beef with the sauce and vegetables, garnished with basil, if desired.

Tips

Active: Forty minutes Slow-cooker time: 4-8 hours

To make ahead: Refrigerate the browned beef (Steps 1-2) and tomato mixture (Step 3) separately for up to one day. Bring the tomato mixture to a boil before adding to the slow cooker.

Equipment: five- to six-quart slow cooker

Nutrition Facts

Serving Size: Three oz. beef & one cup vegetables each

Per Serving: 318 calories; protein 34.7g; carbohydrates 12.8g; dietary fiber 3.1g; sugars 6.2g; fat 10.7g; saturated fat 3.2g; cholesterol 98.9mg; vitamin a iu 6776.9IU; vitamin c 17.4mg; folate 26.3mcg; calcium 69mg; iron 3.5mg; magnesium 36mg; potassium 697.7mg; sodium 538.4mg.

Exchanges: Two vegetable, four and a half lean meat, half fat

- **Cream of Turkey & Wild Rice Soup**

Got leftover cooked chicken or turkey? Cook up a pot of soup! This low-sodium soup recipe is a healthier twist on a classic creamy turkey and wild rice soup that hails from Minnesota. Serve with a crisp romaine salad and whole-grain bread.

Active: Thirty five mins

Total: Thirty five mins

Servings: Four

Ingredients:

One tablespoon extra-virgin olive oil

Two cups sliced mushrooms, (about four ounces)

Three-quarter cup chopped celery

Three-quarter cup chopped carrots

One-quarter cup chopped shallots

One-quarter cup all-purpose flour

One-quarter teaspoon salt

One-quarter teaspoon freshly ground pepper

Four cups reduced-sodium chicken broth

One cup quick-cooking or instant wild rice, (see Ingredient Note)

Three cups shredded cooked chicken, or turkey (Twelve ounces; see Tip)

Half cup reduced-fat sour cream

Two tablespoons chopped fresh parsley

Directions:

Step one

Heat oil in a large saucepan over medium heat. Add mushrooms, celery, carrots and shallots; cook, stirring, until softened, about 5 minutes. Add flour, salt and pepper; cook, stirring, for 2 minutes more.

Step two

Add broth and bring to a boil, scraping up any browned bits. Add rice and reduce heat to a simmer. Cover and cook until the rice is tender, five to seven minutes. Stir in turkey (or chicken), sour cream and parsley; cook until heated through, about two minutes more.

Ingredient note

Quick-cooking or instant wild rice has been parboiled to reduce the cooking time. Conventional wild rice takes forty to fifty minutes to cook. Be sure to check the cooking directions when selecting your rice--some brands labeled "quick" take about thirty minutes to cook. If you can't find the quick-cooking variety, just add cooked conventional wild rice along with the turkey at the end of Step two.

Tip

To poach chicken breasts, place boneless, skinless chicken breasts in a medium skillet or saucepan. Add lightly salted water to cover and bring to a boil. Cover, reduce heat to low and simmer gently until chicken is cooked through and no longer pink in the middle, ten to twelve minutes.

Nutrition Facts

Serving Size: About one and three-quarter cups

Per Serving: 378 calories; protein 36.9g; carbohydrates 28.5g; dietary fiber 2.7g; sugars 2.8g; fat 10.6g; saturated fat 3.7g; cholesterol 79.7mg; vitamin a iu 4518.3IU; vitamin c 6.3mg; folate 57.3mcg; calcium 73.2mg; iron 2.4mg; magnesium 45.7mg; potassium 748.3mg; sodium 364.1mg; thiamin 0.2mg.

Exchanges: One and a half starch, one vegetable, three lean meat, one fat

- **Green Goddess Salad with Chickpeas**

In this cucumber, tomato, Swiss cheese and chickpea salad recipe, a healthy green goddess dressing is made from avocado, buttermilk and herbs. The extra dressing is delicious served with grilled vegetables.

Active: Fifteen mins

Total: Fifteen mins

Servings: Two

Ingredients:

Dressing

One avocado, peeled and pitted

One and half cups buttermilk

One-quarter cup chopped fresh herbs, such as tarragon, sorrel, mint, parsley and/or cilantro

Two tablespoons rice vinegar

Half teaspoon salt

Salad

Three cups chopped romaine lettuce

One cup sliced cucumber

One (fifteen ounce) cans chickpeas, rinsed

One-quarter cup diced low-fat Swiss cheese

Six cherry tomatoes, halved if desired

Directions:

Step one

To prepare dressing: Place avocado, buttermilk, herbs, vinegar and salt in a blender. Puree until smooth.

Step two

To prepare salad: Toss lettuce and cucumber in a bowl with one-quarter cup of the dressing. Top with chickpeas, cheese and tomatoes. (Refrigerate the extra dressing for up to three days.)

- **Ginger-Tahini Oven-Baked Salmon & Vegetables**

The tahini sauce does double duty in this healthy salmon recipe, serving as a glaze for the fish and also as a drizzle for the entire dish at the end of cooking. The green beans are cooked just slightly in this recipe, to still be crisp. If you like your green beans tenderer, look for thinner beans or haricot verts in the grocery store; they'll cook more quickly. This sheet-pan dinner recipe is not only delicious-- it also comes together with just twenty five minutes of active prep time, and there's only one pan to clean up afterwards!

Active: Twenty five mins

Total: Fifty mins

Servings: Four

Ingredients

One large sweet potato, cubed (about Twelve oz.)

One pound white button or cremini mushrooms cut into one-inch pieces (six cups)

Two tablespoons olive oil, divided

Half teaspoon salt, divided

One pound green beans, trimmed

Two tablespoons reduced-sodium soy sauce

One tablespoon plus two tsp. tahini

One tablespoon plus one tsp. honey

One and half teaspoons finely grated fresh ginger

One and one-quarter pounds salmon, preferably wild-caught, cut into four portions

Two teaspoons rice vinegar

Two tablespoons chopped fresh chives (Optional)

Directions:

Step one

Place a large rimmed baking sheet in the oven. Position one rack in the middle of the oven and another about six inches from the broiler. Preheat to 425 degrees F.

Step two

Combine sweet potato, mushrooms, one Tbsp. oil, and one-quarter tsp. salt in a large bowl; toss to coat.

Step three

Remove the baking sheet from the oven. Spread the vegetable mixture in an even layer on the pan; roast, stirring once, until the sweet potatoes are starting to brown, about twenty minutes.

Step four

Meanwhile, toss green beans with the remaining one Tbsp. oil and one-quarter tsp. salt. Combine soy sauce, tahini, honey, and ginger in a small bowl.

Step five

Remove the pan from the oven. Move the mushrooms and sweet potatoes to one side and place the green beans on the other side. Place salmon in the middle, nestling it on top of the vegetables, if necessary. Spread half of the tahini sauce on top of the salmon. Roast until the salmon flakes, eight to ten minutes more. Turn broiler to high; move the pan to the top rack and broil until the salmon is glazed, about three minutes.

Step six

Stir vinegar into the remaining tahini sauce and drizzle it over the salmon and vegetables. Garnish with chives, if desired, and serve.

Tips

To make ahead: Prepare tahini sauce (Step four) up to one day ahead; cover and refrigerate.

Nutrition Facts

Serving Size: One piece salmon plus one and three-quarter cups vegetables

Per Serving: 555 calories; protein 37.7g; carbohydrates 37.3g; dietary fiber 7.6g; sugars 15.6g; fat 29.9g; saturated fat 5.9g; cholesterol 78mg; vitamin a iu 13047IU; vitamin c 21.1mg; folate 112mcg; calcium 102.6mg; iron 2.8mg; magnesium 101.7mg; potassium 1387.7mg; sodium 718.4mg.

Tips

To make ahead: Cover and refrigerate leftover dressing for up to three days.

Nutrition Facts

Serving Size: Two and three-quarter cups

Per Serving: 304 calories; protein 21.7g; carbohydrates 39.8g; dietary fiber 11.9g; sugars 10.1g; fat 7.5g; saturated fat 1.7g; cholesterol 12mg; vitamin a in 6774.1IU; vitamin c 14mg; folate 180.9mcg; calcium 420mg; iron 2.5mg; magnesium 71.8mg; potassium 641.4mg; sodium 465mg.

Exchanges: Two starch, one high-fat protein, one lean protein, one vegetable, half fat.

- **Sheet-Pan Chicken Fajita Bowls**

Skip the tortillas in favor of this warm fajita salad, which features a nutritious medley of chicken with roasted kale, bell peppers and black beans. The chicken, beans and vegetables are all cooked on the same pan, so this healthy dinner is easy to make and the cleanup is easy too.

Active: Twenty mins

Total: Forty mins

Servings: Four

Ingredients:

Two teaspoons chili powder

Two teaspoons ground cumin

Three-quarter teaspoon salt, divided

Half teaspoon garlic powder

Half teaspoon smoked paprika

One-quarter teaspoon ground pepper

Two tablespoons olive oil, divided

One and one-quarter pounds chicken tenders

One medium yellow onion, sliced

One medium red bell pepper, sliced

One medium green bell pepper, sliced

Four cups chopped stemmed kale

One (fifteen ounce) can no-salt-added black beans, rinsed

One-quarter cup low-fat plain Greek yogurt

One tablespoon lime juice

Two teaspoons water

Directions:

Step one

Place a large rimmed baking sheet in the oven; preheat to 425 degrees F.

Step two

Combine chili powder, cumin, half tsp. salt, garlic powder, paprika, and ground pepper in a large bowl. Transfer 1 tsp. of the spice mixture to a medium bowl and set aside. Whisk 1 Tbsp. oil into the remaining spice mixture in the large bowl. Add chicken, onion, and red and green bell peppers; toss to coat.

Step three

Remove the pan from the oven; coat with cooking spray. Spread the chicken mixture in an even layer on the pan. Roast for fifteen minutes.

Step four

Meanwhile, combine kale and black beans with the remaining one-quarter tsp. salt and one Tbsp. olive oil in a large bowl; toss to coat.

Step five

Remove the pan from the oven. Stir the chicken and vegetables. Spread kale and beans evenly over the top. Roast until the chicken is cooked through and the vegetables are tender, five to seven minutes more.

Step six

Meanwhile, add yogurt, lime juice, and water to the reserved spice mixture; stir to combine.

Step seven

Divide the chicken and vegetable mixture among 4 bowls. Drizzle with the yogurt dressing and serve.

Tips

Tip: For easier weeknight prep, slice vegetables the night before; cover and refrigerate.

To make ahead: Prepare spice mixture (Step one) up to two days ahead; store in an airtight container.

Nutrition Facts

Serving Size: Two chicken tenders, one and one-quarter cups vegetables plus generous one Tbsp. sauce

Per Serving: 343 calories; protein 42.7g; carbohydrates 23.7g; dietary fiber 8.2g; sugars 3.8g; fat 9.9g; saturated fat 1.4g; cholesterol 70.9mg; vitamin a iu 2774.9IU; vitamin c 72.9mg; folate 25.3mcg; calcium 187.3mg; iron 3.6mg; magnesium 62.7mg; potassium 579.8mg; sodium 605.1mg.

- **Vegan White Bean Chili**

Fresh Anaheim (or poblano) chiles add mild heat to this classic white bean chili and contribute lots of smoky flavor. Quinoa adds body to the chili, while diced zucchini provides pretty flecks of green and increases the veggie content.

Active: Thirty five mins

Total: One hrs five mins

Servings: six

Ingredients

One-quarter cup avocado oil or canola oil

Two cups chopped seeded Anaheim or poblano chiles (about three)

One large onion, chopped

Four cloves garlic, minced

Half cup quinoa, rinsed

Four teaspoons dried oregano

Four teaspoons ground cumin

One teaspoon salt

Half teaspoon ground coriander

Half teaspoon ground pepper

Four cups low-sodium vegetable broth

Two (fifteen ounce) cans no-salt-added white beans, rinsed

One large zucchini, diced (about three cups)

One-quarter cup chopped fresh cilantro

Two tablespoons lime juice, plus wedges for serving

Directions:

Step one

Heat oil in a large pot over medium heat. Add chiles, onion and garlic. Cook, stirring, until the vegetables are softened, five to seven minutes. Add quinoa, oregano, cumin, salt, coriander and pepper; cook, stirring, until aromatic, about 1 minute. Stir in broth and beans. Bring to a boil. Reduce heat to a simmer. Partially cover and cook, stirring occasionally, for 20 minutes. Add zucchini; cover and continue cooking until the zucchini is soft and the chili has thickened, ten to fifteen minutes more. Stir in cilantro and lime juice. Serve with lime wedges, if desired.

Tips

To make ahead: Refrigerate chili for up to four days. Reheat before serving.

Nutrition Facts

Serving Size: One and one-third cups

Per Serving: 283 calories; protein 9.7g; carbohydrates 36.7g; dietary fiber 8.4g; sugars 6.6g; fat 11.7g; saturated fat 1.3g; vitamin a iu 757.3IU; vitamin c 135.4mg; folate 77.7mcg; calcium 96.4mg; iron 3.9mg; magnesium 107.6mg; potassium 670.7mg; sodium 529.4mg; thiamin 0.7mg.

Exchanges: Two fat, two vegetable, one and half starch, half lean protein

- **Loaded Black Bean Nacho Soup**

Jazz up a can of black bean soup with your favorite nacho toppings, such as cheese, avocado and fresh tomatoes. A bit of smoked paprika adds a bold flavor kick, but you can swap in any warm spices you prefer, such as cumin or chili powder. Look for a soup that contains no more than 450 mg sodium per serving.

Active: Ten mins

Total: Ten mins

Servings: Two mins

Ingredients

One (eighteen ounce) carton low-sodium black bean soup

One-quarter teaspoon smoked paprika

Half teaspoon lime juice

Half cup halved grape tomatoes

Half cup shredded cabbage or slaw mix

Two tablespoons crumbled cotija cheese or other Mexican-style shredded cheese

Half medium avocado, diced

Two ounces baked tortilla chips

Directions:

Step one

Pour soup into a small saucepan and stir in paprika. Heat according to package directions. Stir in lime juice.

Step two

Divide the soup between two bowls and top with tomatoes, cabbage (or slaw), cheese and avocado. Serve with tortilla chips.

Tips

Read more: How to Amp up Canned Soup to Make It a Healthy Meal

Nutrition Facts

Serving Size: about one cup

Per Serving: 350 calories; protein 10.1g; carbohydrates 44.1g; dietary fiber 9.4g; sugars 3.5g; fat 16.9g; saturated fat 3.1g; cholesterol 7.5mg; vitamin a in 860.3IU; vitamin c 19.1mg; folate 52.1mcg; calcium 192.6mg; iron 2.5mg;

magnesium 61.5mg; potassium 351.8mg; sodium 291.4mg; thiamin 0.1mg.

Exchanges: one fat, one starch, one vegetable, half high-fat protein, half lean protein

- **Roast Chicken & Sweet Potato**

Healthy chicken and sweet potato recipes are always a delicious and reliable choice for dinner. This low-calorie sheet-pan meal combines chicken thighs and sweet potatoes and cooks up fast in a very hot oven. Serve with a fall salad of mixed greens, sliced apples and blue cheese.

Total: Forty five mins

Servings: Four

Ingredients

Two tablespoons whole-grain or Dijon mustard

Two tablespoons chopped fresh thyme or 2 teaspoons dried

Two tablespoons extra-virgin olive oil, divided

Half teaspoon salt, divided

Half teaspoon freshly ground pepper, divided

One and half-two pounds bone-in chicken thighs, skin removed

Two medium sweet potatoes, peeled and cut into one-inch pieces

One large red onion, cut into 1-inch wedges

Directions:

Step one

Position rack in lower third of oven; preheat to 450 degrees F. Place a large rimmed baking sheet in the oven to preheat.

Step two

Combine mustard, thyme, one tablespoon oil and one-quarter teaspoon each salt and pepper in a small bowl; spread the mixture evenly on chicken.

Step three

Toss sweet potatoes and onion in a bowl with the remaining one tablespoon oil and one-quarter teaspoon each salt and pepper. Carefully remove the baking sheet from the oven and spread the vegetables on it. Place the chicken on top of the vegetables.

Step four

Return the pan to the oven and roast, stirring the vegetables once halfway through, until the vegetables are tender and beginning to brown and an instant-read thermometer inserted into a chicken thigh registers 165 degrees F, thirty to thirty-five minutes.

Tips

Cut Down on Dishes: A rimmed baking sheet is great for everything from roasting to catching accidental drips and spills. For effortless cleanup and to keep your baking sheets in tip-top shape, line them with a layer of foil before each use.

Nutrition Facts

Per Serving: 408 calories; protein 26.9g; carbohydrates 33.5g; dietary fiber 5.2g; sugars 11.7g; fat 17.4g; saturated fat 3.7g; cholesterol 86.1mg; vitamin a iu 22430.7IU; vitamin c 26.4mg; folate 32mcg; calcium 74.7mg; iron 2.8mg; magnesium 56.5mg; potassium 636.4mg; sodium 554.3mg; thiamin 0.2mg.

Exchanges: One and half starch, one and half vegetable, four and half lean meat, one and half fat

- **Slow-Cooker Chicken & White Bean Stew**

This load-and-go slow-cooker chicken recipe is perfect for a busy weeknight dinner. Serve this Tuscan-inspired dish with crusty bread, a glass of Chianti and a salad.

Active: Fifteen mins.

Total: Seven hrs thirty five mins.

Ingredients:

One pound dried cannellini beans, soaked overnight and drained (see Tip)

Six cups unsalted chicken broth

One cup chopped yellow onion

One cup sliced carrots

One teaspoon finely chopped fresh rosemary

One (Four ounce) Parmesan cheese rind plus two thirds cup grated Parmesan, divided

Two bone-in chicken breasts (1 pound each)

Four cups chopped kale

One tablespoon lemon juice

One-half teaspoon kosher salt

One- half teaspoon ground pepper

Two tablespoons extra-virgin olive oil

A quarter cup flat-leaf parsley leaves

Directions:

Step one

Combine beans, broth, onion, carrots, rosemary and Parmesan rind in a six-quart slow cooker. Top with chicken. Cover and cook on Low until the beans and vegetables are tender, seven to eight hours.

Step two

Transfer the chicken to a clean cutting board; let stand until cool enough to handle, about ten minutes. Shred the chicken, discarding bones.

Step three

Return the chicken to the slow cooker and stir in kale. Cover and cook on High until the kale is tender, twenty to thirty minutes.

Step four

Stir in lemon juice, salt and pepper; discard the Parmesan rind. Serve the stew drizzled with oil and sprinkled with Parmesan and parsley.

Tips

Tip: To save time, you can substitute four (fifteen ounce) cans no-salt-added cannellini beans (rinsed) for the soaked dried beans.

Equipment: six-qt. slow cooker

Nutrition Facts

Serving Size: One and a quarter cups

Per Serving: 493 calories; protein 44.2g; carbohydrates 53.8g; dietary fiber 27.4g; sugars 4.5g; fat 10.9g; saturated fat 3g; cholesterol 67.8mg; vitamin a iu 4792.5IU; vitamin c 20.3mg; folate 31.8mcg; calcium 198.7mg; iron 7.1mg; magnesium 148.9mg; potassium 1556.6mg; sodium 518.4mg.

Exchanges: lean four and one-half protein, two starch, one fat, one vegetable, one-half high-fat protein

Manufactured by Amazon.ca
Bolton, ON

30771811R00048